The Habits Handbook

The Habits Handbook

To Strong, Lean & Healthy

Dr. Laura Sparks

drlaurasparks.com

CONTENTS

Introduction	1
1 ▎ Food is Not Your Friend...	3
2 ▎ Get out of the Rut	9
3 ▎ Re-Define the Clean-Plate	13
4 ▎ Protein & Veggies	19
5 ▎ Give Yourself a Break Today: Intermittent Fasting	25
6 ▎ Success Habits	31
7 ▎ Get Rid of Refined Sugar	37
8 ▎ Alcohol & Your Body, Your Sacred Temple	43
9 ▎ Are You Holding Water?	48
10 ▎ Variety is the Spice of Life	51
CONCLUSION	55
ABOUT THE AUTHOR	56

Introduction

This book is not intended to be a comprehensive tome on all things nutrition & body chemistry. Although I have studied both extensively, this is simply a review of what I see.

I hope to provide effective practical applications, help you to learn to eat to heal your body and to maximize how it performs for you. Ultimately, so that you function well in everyday life.

See, I have had the pleasure of helping real people get healthy for 30 years. As a student of nutrition, I have been geeking out on this stuff for most of my adult life--reading everything I can get my hands on, constantly tuning in to how food affects me and those around me. Always noticing. Constantly learning.

The truth is, it all started with a very real love of food. **I love to eat.** I love all the different flavors and I love tasting *everything*. But more than all of that, I love how even the smallest changes in diet can result in visible changes in how your body looks **and how it will perform for you**. And how, even if you are far from perfect in your execution, your body can *still change for the better and heal.* That's if you choose well and consistently.

What follows is the best of my best, distilled down for you to **workable solutions.**

If you really want to do this, everything is here....to help you get a working understanding of how your food choices might be sabotaging your health. And then to get a strategy to get on with the business of getting well.

Please know that there is **no judgement here.** We are all on our own journey. We all have our own perfect timing. I know that you have been doing the very best that you could possibly do with the information you have been given.

Listen, if you are struggling, you are not alone. It is nothing to be ashamed of. Weight issues coupled with nutritional deficiencies have reached epidemic proportions in the Western world. At a time, ironically, when we have more and better food available than at any other time in history.

And that might actually be part of the problem. So much food, so little time, right? Well, no, not really.

Here is what I know for sure:

It is time to take back our health and to **give the gift of our health** to future generations. No pressure, but your life is depending on it.

Please remember that being magnificently healthy is your God-given destiny; in fact, you were quite literally made for it.

If you 'aren't feelin' it' right now, I am so glad you are here. This is your time.

Welcome home. Welcome back to you.

1

Food is Not Your Friend...

...It is **actually your employee.**

Or should be.

We say things like: I love ice cream, or chocolate or donuts... or (insert your favorite food here).
We are having a one-way love affair with food.

And we are **massively confused.** Food will never love us back. Never, not even for a minute.

In fact, it is quite the opposite, especially when we eat things that hurt us. Americans walk around eating as though their bodies are trash cans with hairy lids! While it seems like we are getting away with that, that is far from true. Poor nutrition will not necessarily call you out at first blush, but it will definitely catch up with you if it is habitual.

Done right, **food can and should work for you.**

Allow me to use a real-life illustration. If you own a business, you may come to love your staff members. You may be super-grateful for all they do for you and your business. You may have wonderful relationships with your employees, and enjoy their company. Many employers have learned the hard way that it is not a good idea to become best friends with your employees. Listen, you can certainly be friendly, but it can sometimes be a big mistake to become besties.

Likewise, food must work *for you.*
Get in the habit of asking: What can this particular food do *for me*? What vitamins and minerals do you offer? Why would I *hire this* and *not that*?

See, in order to *be free* from food addictions, we must first understand **why we have them in the first place.** But most importantly, we are going to break up this lopsided love affair. You may argue that it is too hard...you can't walk away. You certainly can't give up eating, so therefore you will always be addicted.

The truth is, **you don't have to be in bondage to food at all.** You CAN be free.

Now before you argue with me, I want you to know that I have been there. If there was ever a certifiable food addict, it was me. I remember years. Okay, let's get real... *decades,* when food was **all I thought about.** It was the first thing I thought about in the morning and the last thing I thought about before I went to sleep.
Or perhaps more accurately, my weight was the last thing I thought about, as I tentatively ran my hand over my swollen abdomen. I can vividly recall lying in bed at the end of a long and perfectly productive day, thinking about how I had failed myself. Yet again. Wondering exactly how (and then *if*) I might get it right tomorrow. I always believed that I would. Afterall, other people seemed to be able to do this, didn't they?

If all of this sounds familiar, I assure you *there is hope.* As a former food addict, I know this is true.

I know that if I can conquer this addiction, you can too! But it starts with a willingness to let it all go.

Yes. Let's start with just that. Are you willing?

A willingness to start by making the tiniest of changes. A willingness to let go of your tired, ineffective and time-worn patterns that have become habits. The willingness to let food go as your constant companion.

To let go, once and for all, and make room for the new.

The **good news** with habits is that *you can change them.*

But here is the deal. You cannot cling to food as a weird and distant partner...expecting it to do a job that it **cannot** and **will not** ever do for you.

You may think your favorite food brings *comfort* when you are sad, or *engagement* when you are lonely or bored, but the truth is, that you are simply erroneously *believing* those lies! Trust me, it is very easy to do. Remember, I have been there. And yes, I knew better.

One of the hardest things that I put myself through was to continue to be functionally addicted even when I started to understand all the things that I am about to teach you. And just like any addict, I heaped on the guilt and shame. Heaped it on any time that I failed to do all the things that I knew were right.

Here's the thing. When we look to food to do the job of making us feel better. we will always be disappointed. When we need it to do the job of perking us up when we don't get enough rest, for instance. Or, we get pulled into thinking food will help us celebrate special occasions and that it is okay to over-eat if we are celebrating something!

Further, we think that we simply can't leave home without it for any reason. Or, we stop and eat on our way anywhere, because we are convinced we will starve before we arrive or can get back home to the fridge.

In reality, food is only there to feed our bodies. That is the absolute *best* it can do, at the very top of its game. Food's best work is to **simply nourish our bodies.** That's it.

It is not magic.
It is not an emotional healer.
It is not a crutch.
It is not your friend.
Or lover.

Listen, we don't even have to be friends with it.
And contrary to popular opinion, *we don't have to love it!*

In fact, I will tell you a secret: **it might be better for us if we actually don't.** Love it, that is. We may be better off. A good portion of over-eating happens because it "just tastes soooo good", that we think we can't stop. Or we simply don't want to.

Have you ever considered that *one bite* holds all the same great flavor of the whole thing? Digest that one for a moment. **You have the same enjoyment in one or two bites of your favorite food as when you over-indulge.** Maybe even more so.

See, as you learn to honor yourself and your body, those wonderful tastes that you savor can become enjoyable again. It doesn't taste any better to have two pieces of your favorite pie. It doesn't taste any better to eat the entire bag of Oreos. How do I know? I have done it.

I promise you, by the time you get to cookie #24, you are ready to 'lose your cookies!' And yes, I have been there too. See, our bodies recognize (sometimes way before we do, cognitively) when we have too much of a good thing.

For me, I am embarrassed to say, it didn't happen once, but so many times that I actually lost count. I was so addicted to food, so 'in-love' with food, that I could never seem to stop myself from overdoing it.

I would binge eat, fast and furious, and usually alone. While everyone knew that I had a healthy appetite, no one knew how much I would consume in secret. The irony was that the shame of my overconsumption was consuming me. And **not once** did that food *ever* love me back.

When I stuffed myself to what felt like bursting, I would then have to make myself sick (that is, if my body didn't do it first), gaining some immediate physical relief. At times, I would repeat this cycle several times in a day.

I simply couldn't eat enough to get relief from my anxiety, my feelings of inadequacy or my loneliness. Ashamed of my behavior, stuck in this cycle, I felt alone and hopeless.

No, food is not a good lover.

As I began to slowly dig myself out of this dark place, I started with thinking about food as an employee. Just like you would hire *the best,* most qualified, help you can find for your business, I encourage you to hire the best quality food you can afford.

Just like you are not hiring a friend to keep you company at work, you don't have to love your food choice. No, you actually don't. *Not loving* your food might be your first step in getting rid of your addiction, your obsession or your love affair.

Forever.

Listen, **here is a bonus.**

When you break up with food and let go of this love affair, chances are **your real-life human relationships will actually improve.** I dare you to give it a try.

Here's the even better news: **Real people do have the ability to love you back!**

2

Get out of the Rut

Do you remember when your parents made you eat your vegetables? Mine were relentless.

This well-intended nutritional advice helped us to get accustomed to different and unusual tastes. My own mom, God bless her, was definitely NOT a nutritional expert. She believed in sugar and bacon and butter on **everything!** (Still does, by the way.)

Thankfully though, she was not okay with me eating pizza for every meal. I was taught to eat everything on my plate, and yes, even the stuff that was 'gross'. Growing up in the 1940's & 50's, with much food scarcity, she believed in **three square meals a day**, like a religion, and snacks to boot, whether her kids were hungry or not. She believed that food, and lots of it, *is necessary* for the survival of children, no matter what. To this day, and to her credit, she loves to cook and feed people.

And so as a natural result, I learned to eat. I don't think that is a bad thing. While I didn't love it at the time, I will be forever grateful that I learned to at least *try everything*. This has allowed me to develop a very diverse palate, which I have seen to be an important trait of successful weight-losers.

See, we tend to **get stuck in nutritional ruts,** particularly when we are trying to lose weight! Especially when certain foods have 'worked' in the past. In this chapter, we will discuss why they aren't 'working' now.

For example, salads have a reputation of being 'safe' and effective for weight loss. Perhaps when you first started eating salad, you saw the needle move in the right direction. So now you have developed a great salad habit. Great job! Your body legitimately *loves* all those nutrients.

However, often in order to feel full, your salad must be super-sized. And in order for it to taste good, you are drenching it with salad dressings, cheese, croutons. Things that just might be working against you and your weight-loss goals.

There are 3 big problems with this:

1. Commercial salad dressings are either **high in fat and/or sugar** and are basically empty calories.
2. You are **reinforcing the 'need to eat'** behavior with every bite.
3. **Salad is predominately carbohydrate**, so the more we eat, the more we store. That's right, as *fat.* (More on that later).

So, while we think we are doing ourselves a favor with eating the big salad, we might be shooting our weight loss efforts in the proverbial foot. Don't misunderstand, I am a *big fan* of salads, to be sure. But we have to be honest with ourselves. We can't trick ourselves into thinking we are doing better than we are.

See, there is the tendency to think eating salads somehow earns you the right to indulge. I remember my own eating of the big salad *and* the big hunk of bread *and* whatever my husband was having... (who, by the way, almost never ate the salad with me and who *doesn't* struggle with his weight!)

I thought that I earned it, needed the food, and most importantly, **I felt hungry!** Of course I did...

I know now that I *was* hungry. But not for what I thought. I was hungry for a variety of cooked vegetables and protein. I was legitimately hungry for **the nutrition of variety.** The big salad was no longer feeding me what my body most craved. The nutrients were no longer novel.

If this sounds familiar, I am hereby granting you permission to eat something different...
(...You're welcome!)

If you have a well-ingrained 'tried and true' big salad habit, this might be a bit of a challenge for you to break free, but I assure you that your body will thank you. Now is the time to invoke those 'try new things' skills that your parents worked so hard to foster in your childhood. Think of it as **new-found freedom.**

Freedom to choose your food from a **huge variety** of healthy things.
Freedom to **expand** your horizons.
Freedom from the boring, mundane sameness.
Freedom to shed the *excess* weight, which may be a **by-product** of this sameness.

Listen, there is real, scientific evidence that your metabolism actually drops. Evidence that your metabolic rate *slows down,* when you eat the same things always, with little or no deviation. Break free from the monotony *and* boost your metabolism as a bonus.

Here's the thing. We are **excellent adaptors.** So, when you are super-consistent with what you are eating, your body adapts to those foods and doesn't have to work very hard to digest them for energy. This would be why eating that salad may not be 'working' anymore for your weight loss. This is why we tend to plateau. As you begin to 'mix it up', it is like you are waking your body up from a hibernation of sorts. Take a wild guess at what might happen to your energy...

You guessed it. **If your metabolism increases, so does your energy!**

They work hand-in-hand. Always working for you, always doing their best work to keep you healthy and vital. Research done by Lyn-Genet Recitas, wholistic nutritionist and author of The Plan Diet, identified that eating the same stuff on repeat can produce a sort of sensitivity to that food..an actual inflammatory reaction! That chronic inflammation can ultimately end up in **chronic weight gain or inability to shed excess.** (More on her work later... we will delve into inflammatory food in Chapter 8.)

I know it seems hard to believe, but all of this could begin to explain how **your big salad may be making you fat!**

Finally, when you try new things, it takes you out of auto-pilot; you immediately become more conscious and aware of what and how you are eating. This is a very good thing. You tend to slow down and taste your food. The **true upside** of that is that you may naturally *eat less!*

Not only are your meals more interesting, but diversifying your choices will shake up your metabolism, which is critical for fat-burning. More on that later as well, but for now trust me: *It is time* to shake this all up a bit. *It is time* to try new things.

There really is **no downside**...*let's get out of the rut.*

3

Re-Define the Clean-Plate

Let me start by saying that I am not a fan of 'clean-plating'. That is, eating *everything* on your plate, **just because it's there.**

To be clear: There is **no real merit** in eating the whole thing or finishing it all off. No prize, no award, nothing to be gained. Well, except maybe more weight!

I know this sounds harsh, and I surely don't mean it to be. This idea of eating everything that you have portioned yourself may seem like a very noble pursuit and one that has likely been passed down for generations. Initially for our survival and likely from a **place of scarcity**. And listen, in our defense, we come by scarcity honestly.

Our grandparents and even some of our parents knew *real hunger.* Our earlier ancestors have survived economic downturns, famines and even true starvation. Many genuinely remember not knowing where their next meal would come from. And going even further back, the earliest of human kind were obligated to make food-aquistion the whole of their very day-to-day survival.

In the other extreme, I have been told stories of agonizing family dinners, civil 'wars' breaking out within families, when the kids refuse to eat their veggies. Mom and Dad, nutritional vigilantes, insisting that the child must learn to clean his plate. Hereby implying that 'clean-plating' is a skill that must be mastered. And unfortunately that it is somehow wrong to do otherwise.

While there is **a certain merit** in *trying new things* as we learned in the last chapter, force-feeding is almost *never* a good idea. By doing so, especially as children, we lose the ability to identify true satiety (or fullness), and instead we simply learn to eat until it is *all gone.*

Here is the thing, that is a really bad idea when we are talking about the oversized bag of Doritos or box of jumbo donuts. Like an alcoholic who can't leave anything behind in the bottle, so is the addicted eater, who can't leave behind even a tiniest tasty morsel.

Clean-plating was definitely merited in my family and as a good child, I was also proudly described as a *good eater.* That is, I ate anything and everything and yes, all the time. Luckily, when I was 6-10 years old, my metabolism kept pace. This learned behavior caught up with me later of course, as it often does.

When the metabolism slows down in adulthood, coupled with satiety centers that are completely untrained, the inevitable outcome is weight gain. This simple equation is **the cause for much adult obesity** today.

Even more concerning, though, is that children are far more sedentary and the things they eat are far more processed than the average child of a baby boomer. As a result, they are becoming obese far earlier with habits that are *even harder* to change as they get older.

To praise a child simply for cleaning their entire plate or eating it *all*, is invoking an additional dopamine (the feel-good hormone) response in their brains. We have to be really careful how we handle this. They begin to connect that they are *good* when they **finish their food,** and *bad* when they **are not hungry enough to.** So, very early on, we develop strange associations with eating and a weird relationship with hunger.

Here is the truth. Hunger is a **very good thing.** It is a signal to get going and start feeding on something, lest we perish! The lack of hunger is also a very good thing. It tells us that we are fine. It is time to rest, to play, to work or otherwise get on with our lives.

Feeling the difference between hungry and *not* hungry is critical in understanding how to feed yourself and maintain a healthy weight. In developed countries, we are blessed with such an abundance of food that we have all but lost sight of the importance of distinguishing the two.

Feeling hungry is one of the **most wonderful precursors to enjoying a good meal.** Everything simply *tastes better* when you are hungry. The only way to get familiar with the sensation of hunger, is to allow yourself to experience it. Yes, actually experience the feeling.

"But", you may argue, "I hate feeling hungry!"
And I will simply answer, with all due respect, "Why?"

Seriously, though, **why does it bother you?** Why does it have a negative association? Are you actually hungry or just bored? Is it 'time to eat', so like Pavlov's dogs and thei highly conditioned you are simply ready to do so? These are questions to ask yourself as you are thinking about when and what to eat. These are questions to ask when you are deciding to take the next bite or *if you should* clean your plate.

I can actually guess why you dislike hunger, at least partially. You fear the discomfort of hunger **because you are normal.** You fear hunger because it is a biological, life-preserving urge. You fear that you will die if you don't eat...and *right now*. You fear discomfort because you think that you *should feel good* all of the time.

And all of those fears are exactly that.
Fears: False. Evaluations. Appearing. Real.

Rather than cleaning your plate for the sake of it, just because the food is there, let's redefine what a clean plate *actually* is.

I like to think of a clean plate as one that is **free** from chemicals, freshly prepared, jam-packed with nutrients and devoid of empty calories. Clean in the sense of quality. A clean plate is one that we can feel good about consuming, because it fills us up with goodness, not garbage. It moves the nutritional needle forward, fuels the body, and supplies critical building blocks for healing and repair.

The good news is this: **the higher the quality of our food, *the less* we will need or want to eat.** So, while the higher quality might be slightly more expensive, you will also find that you are satiated more efficiently by all of the very effective nutrition. Your cells will signal the hypothalamus (the hunger center in the brain) that it is time to stop eating.

If you don't believe me, **picture this:**

Let's say that you are in the midst of a super busy day and all you have time to gulp down is snack foods...things like pretzels or Doritos or protein bars and fast food. While the protein bar might be a step up, I will guess that you are still feeling hungry (or at the very least, unsatisfied) and craving real food after a day of this.

Let's compare that feeling with how you might feel after consuming the *same* number of calories in the form of a lovely home-cooked meal of lean protein and steamed veggies.

Your body senses the nutrient quality (regardless of the calories) and will either feel *nourished* or feel *hungry*. I would argue in this case, that you aren't really hungry. You simply haven't consumed enough nutrition to signal fullness.

So, *less* really is ***more.*** I challenge you to eat the highest quality of food you can afford. And then stop eating *before* you are full. If you really tune in to your body, you may notice that you are not eating the whole meal. Take a break as you eat, and feel all that goodness in your belly. Drink a bit of water and stop.

There very well may be things left on your plate *and* you will have had enough. And that feeling of *enough,* I promise you, *is very addictive.* (You may even find that this 'feeling of enough' applies to other areas of your life!)

In summary then: Clean-plating...that is, eating everything on your plate for the sake of it... is **not a practice that I recommend.**

And I'm not sure I recommend that you teach it to your kids.

Tuning into your nutritional needs is a *far more accurate way* to determine how much you should be eating. While it may seem like a good thing when we have toddlers, teaching our children to eat everything on their plate, can start them barreling down a very serious slippery slope. A slope of habitual over-eating that they may never claw their way back up from.

Over-riding our personal sensations of satiety **can lead to a lifetime of not being in tune** with our own integrity....Never quite knowing when enough is *really* enough. And that, my friend, will definitely spill over into other areas of our lives.

I don't blame my mom or my upbringing for my eating disorder. I don't think I ever did. Now that I understand why and how I got into this very dangerous loop, I am able to rise above it, catch myself in the act and over-ride my urges.

There were many factors of not-enoughness that I struggled with. I think that I was self-soothing with my chronic binge-eating, then hyper-controlling the consequences with purging. While not the sole cause, suffice it to say: I *do* think that *eating until it is gone* was causal. At least in part.

If you aren't convinced yet, my final argument against 'eating it all gone' arises from practicality. As a mom and the chief cook in my house, I love leftovers. Yes, **love** them.

I can spruce them up, add things in and have lovely meals in minutes. See, if you leave a little behind, every time you eat, you will have the beginnings of your menu for tomorrow. It also gives me the very satisfying feeling of being prepared ahead of time...double bonus!

So, get in the practice of **leaving a little behind**, get in the habit of listening to your body. And you will be amazed at how much less food you are consuming.

Sit back, enjoy the feeling of 'just enough', then get out there and do something fun with your extra time.

Eating might just be over-rated as recreation anyway!

4

Protein & Veggies

It really is that simple.

Here is a mantra that you can chant in your mind if you need help simplifying:

If it is not Protein, it is Carbohydrate or Fat.

Most of the food we consume falls into the broad category of carbohydrate composition. In general, carbs are the snacky things and a good portion of fast food. It also includes fruits and vegetables.
There really is nothing else. For real.

That's it: **Proteins, Carbs and Fats.**
Nutrition 101. Done.

"Okay," You may be saying. "So it might be simple, but it *ain't easy*!" And until this practice becomes a habit, that may be true. However, there is no reason to overcomplicate things unnecessarily.
Furthermore, it really doesn't have to be hard. Believing it can and will be both simple and easy will give you an edge. Remember, what you believe you can do is exactly you will manifest. Believe in your own ability to do this. That starts with simplicity.

Let's get into the nitty-gritty of the protein-carb balance and why it is so important. By attaining some understanding, you can begin to put things into practice and then begin to really shed some pounds.

Proteins are the **building blocks of living tissue.** That is, we need protein to grow and develop, but we also need it for adequate repair and healing.

Not only that, but we need protein to manufacture large molecules, like hormones and enzymes. And while this is critical for growth and development, this is an ongoing need throughout our lifetime. When you don't have enough protein to work with, all of your body's systems are at risk of compromise. Hormone systems, tissues and cells (the basic units of human life) simply *cannot and will not* work properly without adequate protein. Why not, you may ask?

Not only do things 'not work right', but tissues, **cells and organs begin to break down and even begin to fail.** You get sick or have unseen disease processes that begin to consume and overtake your body. Yes, the very body that you are living in, this temple that you reside in and are depending on cannot work if it doesn't have adequate resources to perform all the necessary functions of life.

Understand that the process of breakdown is slow and often unseen. It will rob other tissues of their nutrition and compromise as long as it can before it fails. But, I promise you, there is no way around this. Your body will not be denied.

So clearly, you must get enough protein. Your body is smart enough to begin to consume your own tissues (not fat, by the way) but organs and tissues, when it is deficient in protein. If it doesn't have what it needs to fully re-build your tissue, it will get what it needs one way or the other.

Sometimes the compromise comes in the form of **being 'stingy' with healing processes**. That is, you don't fully recover from a cold or flu and catch the next thing that comes your way. Or that ache or pain from a fall or injury never seems to resolve. Always feeling a little sick or tired or 'just not feeling right' can be your body desperately trying to get your attention.

You guessed it, this is not fun and definitely not healthy. And no, we don't really want to lose weight this way. While a vegetarian, vegan diet or plant-based *is* admirable and has a host of inherent benefits, getting enough protein with these diets can be a very real challenge.

On the flip side then, *with enough protein* in the mix, your body will have all the **amino acids** necessary to maintain a well-functioning body. It will be able to heal and repair constantly, consistently and completely. Healing is such an important part of your weight loss journey that I promise you, it is worth the time you will invest to do this right.

When your body begins to get healthy through adequate exercise and good nutrition, the body will begin to shed the extra weight. Like magic. There will be a reorganization of your body composition that will require that healing and repair is firing on all cylinders. This is the best and safest way **to lose weight permanently.**

What is protein, then?

Meat, fish, chicken, nuts, beans, legumes, seeds, eggs, dairy and parts of whole grain foods are the primary sources of protein in our diet. An egg has 7 grams on average, while 3 ounces of meat will range between 20-25 grams depending on the type of meat and its density. One ounce of cheese or nuts carries about 7 grams, while a half-cup of hummus will pack about 10 grams. This gives you a basic idea, but there are plenty of charts and resources online that I encourage you to reference to get familiar with your favorite sources.

We need about 36% of our body weight in grams of protein every day. So, if you weigh in at 100 lbs, that would be 36 grams of protein required on any given day. Most of us, unless we really focus on it, simply don't get enough. What often if we don't meet that requirement is that we have an insatiable appetite for any and all carbs to fuel our 'gas tank'. The majority of the time, then, if we are not eating enough protein, we are compensating by eating almost anything else. And usually in excess.

I urge you to **get a protein chart** and post it where you can easily see it. A chart that clearly shows you the protein source with the actual grams it provides. Then, begin to watch how you feel as you consume more protein. You will probably surprise yourself.

There is a certain magic that happens when we feed our body **with rich sources of protein**. Nestled in the center of your brain lies a little gland called the hypothalamus. This gland is primarily responsible for triggering and regulating several hormone systems in your body. One of its primary jobs is to signal hunger AND satiety.

Not only is the hypothalamus 100% dependent on protein to ensure that it has the building blocks to perform necessary functions, but it takes its cues directly from protein *when deciding if you have had enough to eat*. See, if you aren't getting enough protein, the hypothalamus won't get the memo. You will constantly feel hungry and continue to eat.

This is why **Atkins and Keto-type diets work.** This is also why the 10 oz steak is so filling. If you have dabbled in a predominantly protein diet, you may have already discovered all the benefits that come with high-protein eating. You may have also discovered that you cannot possibly eat protein 24/7. And this is the good news.

See, your body also needs all the goodness that only fruits and veggies bring to the table. Essential vitamins and nutrients must be in adequate supply to prevent a host of conditions and diseases. You simply cannot afford to live without your veggies.

To simplify, then, **everything that is not protein will serve as fuel.** Literal gas in your 'gas tank'. Carbs and fats will never turn into protein. Their chemistry is completely different. But we need both in our diet to ensure that our body has everything it needs to function well.

While you cannot transform carbs into protein, you body *does* have the ability to turn carbs into fat. All carbs and fats that you don't digest and burn for fuel within a few short hours are stored as fat for a rainy day. This is your body *functioning normally*. This is actually **your body doing it right!**

I often hear people voicing their frustration over their own inability to lose weight. More specifically, complaining that everything they eat goes *straight* to their belly or their hips.

If this is the case for you, the truth is that you have become a very effective *fat-storer*. We train our body to function according to its most relevant needs. When you eat more than you use, *at any given time*, during the day, your body senses this excess and turns on all the hormones that will help you store the extra.

So if you want to lose the weight, if you want to get rid of your fat, the only way you can do this is to burn that fat as fuel. And the only way you can burn your own fat as fuel, is to *stop eating* carbs long enough for your body to feel and sense the deficit.

In other words, when your body senses the need for fuel, in real time, it will trigger the systems that will burn your fat. When your body senses the need, it turns on the glucagon, the hormone that will help you burn your own fat. Remember, **glucagon cannot** *and will not work* **when insulin is in the house.** There is no way around it, you simply **have to take a break** from eating.

If you want to lose weight, specifically fat, you must get your body into fat-burning mode. And you do that by *not eating*. That is, doing something other than eating *for hours* at a time.

Get out of the kitchen.
Stop dragging food with you wherever you go.
Stop stopping everything for a 'needed' snack all day long.

You don't need it. Not all the time anyway.
Give your body a break. Feel that healthy hunger.
Your body is actually yearning for some downtime. There is simply no other way.

Then, do it again tomorrow.
Soon **your body will begin to look different.**

I promise.
Just try it.

5

Give Yourself a Break Today: Intermittent Fasting

As we learned in the last chapter, one of the most powerful ways to get into fat-burning mode is to stop eating. Seems too simple?

Well, maybe that's why it is **so overlooked.**

Here's the deal. There are 2 hormone systems that we touched on that are constantly at work in your body, doing the work of digesting, metabolizing, and converting food to energy:

Insulin, the fat-storing system, and **Glucagon,** the fat-burning system.

Insulin **converts the sugar** you eat into **usable energy.** And then, **stores the excess as fat.**

So, if you do not use 100% of the carbs that you take in, at any given time, your body goes to work storing the excess as fat.

'Over-carbing' causes the insulin system to predominate. When you are giving your body a never-ending supply of carbs, the insulin system is not only in high gear, but it is very **well-adapted to metabolizing sugar** and **storing the excess.** Your body's insulin system is finely-tuned and is now trained to be very efficient in the process of storing fat.

Glucagon, on the other hand, only gets to come to work **when sugar is in short supply.** That is, glucagon can only work in the state of **low blood glucose.** Your body senses its need for energy and sends glucagon in, to **release energy *from* your stored fat.**

It is super-important to understand that the work of the 2 systems is **mutually exclusive.**

That means you cannot have *both* working at the same time. **It is one or the other.** Only when insulin is not at work can glucagon begin the work on your fat cells. That is, the critical work of releasing valuable stored energy, by consuming your very own fat.

In other words, you can only burn your own fat when *insulin is absent.* This is the principle behind **intermittent fasting** *as a vehicle* **for weight loss.**

You are either an efficient fat-burner or an efficient fat-storer, based on your body's adaptation. Remember, this is your body's adaptation to *how you eat.* If you are feeling like everything you eat sticks to you, your insulin or fat storage system is functioning very efficiently. If that is the case, please do not despair. Your body is doing **exactly what is was designed to do.** Nothing has gone wrong.

This is actually very good news: **Your body can be trained to become more efficient** at burning fat for fuel! It just needs a little practice. It is important, however, to remember that it won't get any practice if you never give it a chance to try.

Taking breaks from eating, that is, extended breaks away from carbs specifically, is the simplest way to trigger fat-burning.

I suggest starting with stretching the hours between meals. That is, no more snacking or grazing between meals. This allows glucagon to kick in and do its thing instead, busting up the fat for fuel, at least on a micro-level.

Even the teeniest bite of any carbohydrate (yes, even salad or a carrot!) interrupts the cycle and stops the fat-burn. It doesn't matter how many calories your little bite delivers. That tiny bite takes you from fat-burning to fat-storing mode.

This explains why, even though you may be working super hard in the gym and limiting how much you eat...**your insulin system is out-performing your glucagon system**, you are still gaining or not losing weight.

The solution? Stop snacking, stop grazing.
Yes, stop it.

The goal is to **extend the time between meals** and let your fat-burning system get used to doing some work. Like any other system or process in your body: If you don't use it, *you lose it*.

Fat-burning is no different. If you haven't been using it, you may be losing it.

On the other hand, the more often you allow a fasting state, that is, the more often you stop eating and force your body to use its own resources to find another source of fuel, **the more fat-burning you will do**. And the more often you do that, the more efficient your fat-burning or glucagon system will become.

So, you can and **will become a finely-tuned and efficient fat-burner.**

I know this may seem way over-simplified. I promise you, it *really is* that simple. I have seen it happen over and over again. And so have you. I'll bet you can group most of the people you know as fat-burners or fat-storers. All those 'skinny' people, the thin ones, who won't gain a pound, no matter what they eat or when. They are efficient *fat-burners*.

And then, there are those, perhaps you are one of them, that no matter what you do, you can't stop gaining or can't seem to lose a pound. Efficient *fat-storers*.

Remember, each system works independently and **there no tricks.** That is the good news! It is predictable and reliable. If you stop eating, your body will learn how to burn its own fat as fuel.

Once you realize how important it is to take breaks from eating (and the longer the better) we can begin to implement intermittent fasting.

Intermittent fasting will do 3 primary things for your body:

1. Allow your digestive system a much-needed rest, which will make it *more efficient and more functional.*
2. Allow your liver and kidneys to adequately detox, making them *more functional.*
3. Produce a true fasting state, which will **trigger glucagon and the fat-burning system.**

Here is a **simple example** of how you might make this system work for you.

Complete your last meal of the day by 6 pm and drink only water or herbal tea until bedtime. In the morning, start your day with 10 ounces of lemon water, prolonging your fast for as long as you can. Black coffee or tea is permissible until you break your fast at lunchtime, 11 am-12 pm.

This is a net 17-18 hour fast, time enough to put you into fat-burning, that is, consuming your own body fat for fuel. Keep this up with some regularity and **you are well on your way** to training your body to burn its own fat for fuel.

At the beginning, you may experience some benign light-headedness, hunger pangs, and urges. While this may be a bit uncomfortable, in most cases, it is **totally normal.** The more trained you are at fat-burning, the less frequently you will have those types of symptoms and the easier it will become.

Listen, please remember, if you are burning fat, you are not going hungry. You may feel hungry or think you need food. You **are not going hungry**, you are merely consuming your own previously-stored food sources.

Your body is not the least bit saddened by this. It stored that excess food *for such a time as this.* You can rest assured that it is actually relieved that you finally got the message! You have gotten around to using what's in storage. If you are more than a few pounds overweight, you have lots to consume. **So relax and get busy.**

Need more good news? **Research backs this up.**

To re-cap, your digestive system needs full-stop breaks throughout the day to rest and fully rejuvenate to function at its best. You actually need a fat-burning system that works well to eliminate the fat stores and the toxicity that is stored within. So this my friend, is a win-win.

Furthermore, we know that people who carry lower overall body weight and BMI live longer and have more energy, stronger immunity, and higher net worth. Okay, okay, I made up the net worth thing to see if you are paying attention. But then again, if you are eating less, spending less on health care costs, feeling better, more energized…it is more than probable that you will have more money. Bonus.

In summary, then: *Drop the snacking* and grazing and *extend the periods of time* between meals. And you will truly be off to the races…**And burning your own fat as fuel!**

6

Success Habits

Habits are truly where the rubber meets the road.

Our *choices* determine *our habits* and **our habits create our reality.**

For good or for bad, the quality of our life comes down to what we choose to do on a *daily* basis.

So, what we repeatedly *d*o today will determine the success of our outcomes. And then, what we repeatedly do tomorrow, and the next day will create our very life. I know that seems overly simplistic, but **success is really just that simple.**

How many times do you catch yourself **eating simply out of habit**? I often find I am famished (or conditioned) to eat at certain times, that I will catch myself snacking unconsciously, just because it is *that* time of day. I catch myself on a snacking frenzy around 12 pm and then again at 5 pm. My appetite seems to ramp up, can even become insatiable at times and I catch myself eating **everything in my path.**

Here's an example: I caught myself in the very act of this a few months ago...eating and preparing food the minute I walked in the door. I hadn't even taken my coat off! Ridiculous, I know. Everybody in the house was hungry, including me. I didn't have a minute to spare, or so I thought. I simply got right to it.

As I took a step back and realized what I was doing, I literally laughed out loud, only to realize I was crying on the inside. So conditioned to eat at a certain time, so famished, I dove right in, with little to no conscious thought. This is *not* the way to do it, but at least I am learning to observe and catch myself in the act.

I am also learning that it feels way **more serene**, way less stressful and less 'put-upon,' to be in comfortable, non-work clothes. Yes, my family and I can wait the few minutes it takes to change into something more comfortable. Not one of us will perish if I take those few moments.

Here is another example. I usually eat lunch around noonish. From my earliest memories as a child, to years of taking a consistent lunch time at the clinic, I simply get hungry around noon. So, even if I have a late breakfast, I am ready to eat around 12 pm, whether I am hungry or not. Clearly, if I eat a brunchy-type breakfast at 11 am, I don't need to be eating again at noon!

It is not that I can't break these habits. There are definitely times when I am forced to work through lunch or something else 'up-ends' my usual lunchtime. There are times when I am forced to wait until 1 or even as late as 2 pm. If distracted enough, I can survive. I have proven that I don't *have to eat at noon.* However, without an active distraction, with nothing to keep my mind off it, food is what I naturally think about at 12 pm.

In the case where I may have eaten a large breakfast or brunch, later than usual, I can consciously capture my lunch-grubbing thoughts and reason with them.

So it with you. I challenge you to really look at your habits and your habitual feeding times. Your times may be different than those above, but chances are, you are conditioned to eat habitually as well. There is nothing inherently wrong with that, unless you go unconscious in the process. As you create new habits, once of our goals will be to eat very consciously. That is, becoming very aware of your **need for food and nutrition** And ONLY eating for that reason.

Here's what you could truthfully say back to your own mind, when you are tempted to over-eat:

"You just ate. Feel the fullness in your stomach."
"You are not hungry, you couldn't possibly be."
"You are simply habituated. You will have dinner today, later dear. Not now."
"You are fine. You will not die by not eating lunch right now."
"You will be just fine. More than fine."

Learn to observe yourself in your habitual behaviors and be willing to break those habits if necessary. Start by extending the time between meals. That means, crack down on snacking. Try intermittent fasting by eliminating **all snacks.** Y

Yes, there is merit in teaching yourself to go *without food* for extended periods of time.

You can start by eating at a different time, changing your habits on purpose. This has been shown to cause a metabolic boost, simply because it is different.

Every time your body has to adapt to something new, **your metabolism is shaken up and rises to the occasion.**

Next, take steps to extend your night-time fast by pushing the 'breaking of your fast' later or skipping breakfast altogether. Before you know it, you will be fasting for 17-18 hours per day and well on your way to becoming a competent and efficient fat-burner!

Listen, this goes for your grocery habit too.

Don't buy what you have always bought, just because that is what you have always done.

I challenge you to 'eat outside the box'. Maybe it's a healthy new veggie that you have never tried before. New and interesting spices make everything taste better and different. **Enjoy more variety. Get out of your nutritional ruts.** Make the switch to real food and begin to experience the delight.

Remember, simply by mixing it up, you are **triggering your metabolism to run higher.** Any time your body is forced to adapt to something new, your *metabolism will rise* to the occasion.

This is your **official permission slip to try a wide variety of healthy foods.** Foods that you may have been afraid of or hesitant to try. Yes, even if it seems expensive. You are **more than worth it.**

As you shake up your patterns and eating habits, you will be surprised at how easy it really is to adapt to new things. **Change begets change.** As you switch up the pattern and timing of your meals, it will be a natural transition to radically change the types of foods you are eating. Your body might be a bit shocked, but I assure you, your body **will love you** for it!

Just as well-ingrained bad habits can work against us, the **good ones can also work very much for us.**

That is, when good habits are carefully-crafted and we are disciplined enough to stay the course, they will anchor us to a **brand new lifestyle.** Those new habits can begin to shape your life and ultimately your health. Soon you will not recognize yourself!

James Clear, in [Atomic Habits: An Easy & Proven Way to Build Good Habits & Break Bad Ones,](#) shows how it is possible to **skew the game in our favor.** To arrange our lives so that much of what we do becomes automatic. And thereby does not require any discipline at all.

Here's a simple example:

In order to stay on track with my daily water intake, I need to drink 16 ounces of lemon water in the morning. This is not something that I necessarily *want* to do. I like water, but I seriously love my coffee.
I decided to commit to doing this before I drink my morning coffee or have any breakfast. To make it easier, I refrigerate that tall glass of water before I go to bed, *the night before.* I can simply squeeze the lemon in on demand.

Since I love my morning coffee and I almost never skip this, I realized I could link these two together.
That is, *no coffee* until I have drunk my first 16 ounces of life-giving water.
When linked together, it makes it a no-brainer. It makes me even *want to.*

Here is another one.

I make my lunch ahead of time. Even if I am coming home for lunch, it is pre-made so that when I walk in the door, it is ready in an instant. On the days when I *don't have* something **pre-done or pre-**

planned, I find it way harder to stick to my commitment of eating real food. Way easier to stop for fast food on the way home or eat empty, carby snacks while I figure out or prepare my meal. Listen, it is not impossible, but simply not *skewed* for success.

Similarly, if the rest of my family is eating pizza, I can easily succumb to the peer pressure. That is, unless I have something *ready to go*, or at least an idea of a healthy and delicious alternative. So, when they have pizza, I eat my favorite roasted veggies with all my favorite spices. I outdo the pizza in aroma and flavor every time.

In review:

1. Reduce the steps to your own great food everywhere you can.
2. Cultivate minimal friction for your new habits.
3. Remember, change is fun, adventurous and exciting.
4. **Don't forget to enjoy the journey.**

7

Get Rid of Refined Sugar

Let me start this chapter by reminding you of this: There is no health benefit, or any real nutrition at all, in refined sugar. No, sugar is not one of the food groups. And no, it is not necessary for a well-balanced diet.

We don't need dessert with every meal and we can live without it. We actually can live better without it.

Get this: **We eat more sugar in an average day** than our earliest ancestors ate over the course of a year. I promise you, humans can survive *without* refined sugar.

There are 4 primary things I want you to be aware of regarding this seemingly harmless habit of eating refined sugar:

1. Sugar functions like a drug and can lead to other more serious addictions.
2. Due to the trigger of your insulin response...the more you eat, the more you want.
3. Consuming sugar can produce an adrenal response.
4. Sugar metabolism causes a roller-coaster effect on both energy and mood.

Let's break down each item by taking a closer look. Please know that there is no judgement here. You are not addicted because you are weak or gluttonous. Understand that there are built-in systems in your body that keep you eating the sugar *and keep you addicted.*

1. Sugar functions like a drug.

Sugar is a powerful trigger of our dopamine or feel-good receptors, so technically a drug. These are the same receptors in the brain that respond to morphine and cocaine. And this is what makes sugar so addictive.

So, while you may think you are simply drawn to the great taste, I assure you, there is much more to it than just that. Any time those receptors are triggered and you feel good, you are programming your brain and body to want more. It is built into the very system.

The more you eat, then, the more you want. Not only *in the moment* but over time. We are constantly seeking ways to trigger those receptors and like any drug, we need a larger dose to trigger them. And we constantly seek a larger hit. Just like a cocaine addiction, we continually seek a higher high. This translates into more sugar consumption.

According to Kathleen DesMaisons in <u>Little Sugar Addicts,</u> there is evidence that sugar use (and abuse) at early ages in children leads to a higher likelihood of drug use and abuse later in life. Just know that while your sugar habit seems harmless, it is anything but. Remember, our kids *will do what we do* and *not what we say.*

2. Sugar is an Insulin-trigger: The more you eat, the more you want to eat.

As we have learned previously, when insulin is present, glucagon **cannot work**. That is, any time sugar is in your blood stream (from eating carbs), insulin is working to lower blood sugar and process the ingested sugar. That means fat-burning stops and fat-storing begins.

So, the minute you put a sugary snack in your mouth, **the insulin response is on its way.** Insulin, remember, stores fat instead of burning it. Insulin also increases appetite.

When insulin is present, we want to eat more. And, we inevitably do. The more refined the sugar, the quicker this response. Remember, this response occurs with the consumption of any carbohydrate.

Listen, we have a huge array of amazing fruit choices that don't have that same *rapid glycemic shift.* They are sweet and delightful and pack a beneficial and nutritious punch. However, the more you eat of the refined stuff, the less you want of the not-so-refined, or the healthier fruit-source choices.

We become so habituated to eating the highly-refined sugary things, the lower glycemic options can seem very hum-drum and not at all palatable. That is, they just don't taste good or give us the same zing.

Our tendency to stick with the highly-refined quick delivery sugars is largely *habit-based*. But remember, we *can* change our habits.

Okay, do you need some good news? The reverse is also true.

The less you eat, the less you want. If you can get out of the habit of eating refined sugar, that is, eliminate it from your diet, you will find that you no longer have the drive to eat it at all!

The truth is, people who don't eat sugar on a regular basis find that they **no longer have an appetite for it.** That's right, you lose the taste for all that sugary 'goodness'!

Not only does it no longer taste good to you, but you shift your actual biochemistry and hormone balance. When you don't set yourself up for a rapid sugar response, you no longer find yourself needing it. Your body is simply no longer habituated to it.

3. Consuming sugar can cause an adrenal response.

There is evidence that the negative effect of refined sugar can put such a strain on the human body that **we mount an adrenal or stress response** to it. Adrenaline and cortisol give us energy, they boost our mood, focus, and alertness.

All of that *feels great* in the moment. This is part of why we get a quick energy boost. The reality is that our system is so stressed *by* this chemical assault, that it triggers an emergency response! Yes. To the sugar.

Listen, we have enough stress in our day-to-day lives, we definitely don't need to add to our body's stress with our eating. While this feels great in the moment, the boost is temporary at best.

The pendulum swing in blood sugar and the **resultant *downward spiral* of energy** is definitely not a movement in the right direction nor is there a net increase of energy. The net result is actually a down-cycling of our energy and of course, the immediate need for more sugar. Quite literally, almost as soon as the chemical storm has died down, we reach for another stimulant to increase the dopamine in the brain. The addiction process in a nutshell.

As a result, we **overload our adrenal glands** repeatedly and they will eventually burn out or succumb to adrenal fatigue. This can lead to hormonal disruption, secondary diseases, and long term health problems. These effects can be so slow and insidious that they are almost undetectable. Suffice it to say, the adrenal response in the short term is simply not worth it.

4. Sugar metabolism causes a roller-coaster effect on both energy and mood.

The energy 'roller-coastering' that follows the dramatic swings in blood sugar **can also affect our moods** in a similar way. So, instead of constant, sustained energy and mood, we experience dramatic swings. The tendency to feel angst, anxiety, and even full-on depression can often follow the rapid swings in blood sugar. This comes on so subtly that we often don't even realize that it's happening. You may not even recognize the changes until they are well-advanced, and you are very addicted to your sugar habit.

Patients report a dramatic shift in energy and mood when they give up sugar. It is one of those things that creeps up on us so subtly that we don't realize how bad it has gotten until it is better.

Give yourself a chance to come back to the real you. You might be pleasantly surprised at how cool you are!

As I wrap up my tirade on sugar, there is **one more thing** I would like you to consider. The very first taste of your favorite food *is always as good* as the whole thing. In fact, arguably, the first taste is *even better* than eating the whole thing. And without the guilt to go along with it!

So, if you must eat the sugar, try to **indulge in the teeniest of little tastes.** My grandma taught me this by example and I have followed this principle every since.

I will never forget the fun of going to the dessert table and giggling with delight when we would return with *one of each treat!* But understand, this plate of goodies was collected for the *entire table to share.* My grandma was never overweight and *never* ate **all the treats.**

Maybe I inherited her penchant for tiny tastes or maybe it was learned, I will let you be the judge. All I can tell you for sure is that I love my tiny tastes and it has served me well. I rarely eat the whole thing and without fail, find that the itty bitty tasting of everything is very satisfying indeed.

    I encourage you to at least try this. You may find that with time, like me, that **giving in to the urge is just not worth it.**
    Please remember that each time you do, you are moving yourself from fat-burning to fat-storing. You may find that you don't want to sacrifice **all the good work you are doing all day long**, simply for the sake of that short burst of taste or supposed energy.

    Perhaps with time, you will further see that **the best reward you can give yourself** is staying on your protocol and **continuing along the healing journey** towards your ideal weight.

8

Alcohol & Your Body, Your Sacred Temple

You only have one body on this earth and how you treat it will determine how it will perform for you.

Yes, it is sacred and **valuable beyond measure.**

It will never cease to amaze me how well the human body functions *in spite* of how poorly we fuel it. We would never think to 'feed' our cars as badly as we feed ourselves. And yet, we seem to persist in these habits in spite of knowing better.

While junk food might make you feel good *temporarily*, let me remind you this type of euphoria can only be **temporary**. When we are talking about alcohol, **even more so**. For those who partake, please know that there is no judgment here. I honestly don't think there is anything inherently wrong with having the occasional alcoholic beverage.

Just know that there can be some big consequences to your health and inherent challenges to maintaining your ideal weight when you consume alcohol on a regular basis.

Here are just a few consequences from alcohol use:

1. Long-term alcohol use and abuse can cause permanent brain damage.
2. Your liver has the burden of processing and detoxing.
3. You are effectively mainlining sugar. (Sorry...it's true!)
4. Oh yes...ingesting alcohol will take you out of fat burning.
5. The more you drink, the more you want.

So, let's briefly dive into each one of the above effects and then you can decide if it is still worth it to you.

Like the discussion on sugar, I am not going to strong-arm you to quit, but I will make you aware of what you are doing to your body.

1. Long-term alcohol use and abuse can cause brain damage.

Not only does it impair you in the moment, but the effect on the brain can be long-term and **sometimes irreversible**. Brain damage has been shown to occur at all levels of alcohol consumption.

While it might seem like one of those things that happens to *everyone else and not you,* I assure you that the chemistry of alcohol is **no respecter of persons**. In other words, these devastating effects can happen to anyone.

Of course, this depends on the quantity you consume and the time it takes you to consume it. There is **evidence of long-term brain effects** with the even smallest consumption levels. Particularly, if we drink a lot all at one time. The bottom line, then? No matter how socially accepted and common this practice is: Proceed with caution.

2. Your liver has the burden of processing and detoxing.

We deal with a host of toxicity every day and in so many ways. Pollution, chemicals in our food, drugs, and alcohol are all processed through this hard-working organ. Therefore, overuse and abuse of alcohol can cause chronic liver disease.

An overworked liver can be a **primary cause of weight gain**. This can significantly slow the process of weight loss. We burn and process fat directly through the liver, so it is imperative that this organ is functioning at its best to optimize this function.

Please consider this: All the foreign substances that you ingest **process through the liver.** There is no other way, no other path. This process can be exhausting for the body and organs as they do this work for you. Listen, give them a break. They will thank you by being more efficient. And yes, this will help you lose weight!

3. You are mainlining sugar.

If you take a look at the chemical composition of alcohol, you will see that it is *mostly sugar*. As a fermented product, this is a direct by-product of the fermentation process, so there is no way around this. As a liquid, no chewing is involved and no breakdown required for your body to make it usable for energy. The glycemic index, then, is very high and produces a high glycemic state immediately.

And no, there is **no inherent nutritional value in this suga**r. It absolutely is empty calories and yes...

4. Oh yes...drinking alcohol takes you out of fat-burning.

As we have learned and by now hopefully observed, when there is sugar present in the blood, we are in the business of fat-storing. And remember, any time we are storing fat, we *cannot and will not* burn fat.

I don't know about you, but I really like to eat! I love the taste of food, the textures, the chewing, the swallowing and engaging in the entire process. So, I don't want to sacrifice any opportunity to eat, or waste those precious calories on a drink.

Once again, I will not tell you what to do, but I will warn you to **proceed with caution.**

5. **The more you drink, the more you want.**

Some sources consider alcoholism and your addiction to be on an ongoing continuum. That is, from your first drink, you are **on your way towards alcoholism**.
I know, that sounds extreme and maybe even a bit harsh, but there is much evidence to support this. For some of us, the taste is repugnant. Or perhaps, our memories of the drunken binges of family members is enough to turn us off and head off alcohol abuse at first pass. For others, moderate drinking might fit just fine into their lifestyle. They enjoy the odd drink and have no devastating consequences, addiction-wise. For still others, the first drink sets them on a path that they will never reverse or recover from. And this continuum allows for individuals to fall anywhere in between.

Once again, we are triggering the **feel-good or dopamine receptors** in the brain and habitual use can wreak havoc within our dopamine systems. The more you engage in the business of triggering your dopamine systems, the stronger they get. That is, the neurological connections that control the behavior actually get stronger and more tethered and as a result, you are more addicted.

Please realize that you don't need these substances to be happy. There is an infinite number of activities that can provide real-life fun (and natural healthy dopamine!)

Ultimately, **your happiness comes from within**, never from an external source. When we seek happiness from an external source, it will always be a dead-end street. Learning that one principle will change your life.

Food for thought:

What **healthy sources of happiness** can I engage in that do not involve food or alcohol?

I encourage you to **invest time & energy** in cultivating those things.

9

Are You Holding Water?

Wait, wait, don't tell me. Before you answer this question, I will take the liberty to answer for you. The answer is an unequivocal 'yes'! Of course you are holding water, your body is 70% water. When we don't have adequate supply or simply don't hydrate, **our bodies will hang on to every ounce.**

Our joints will stay swollen and uncomfortable, our fingers and toes might be puffy, our feet hurt when we stand for too long, our eyes have saddlebags. All this, because **we aren't drinking *enough*.** And remember, that is straight up, plain old water, nothing added to it.

We also hold excess water in the form of inflammation, when we eat food that does not agree with us or that we have a subclinical sensitivity to. Over time, this can lead to a **chronic inflammatory condition.**

Lyn-Genet Recitas has developed a super-practical protocol for eliminating diet-induced inflammation in The Plan Diet. While there are others that have done work in this area, her wholistic nutrition approach is genius. Her understanding and experience in this is second to no one.

If you think you are harboring chronic inflammation, which can manifest in 'unlosable weight', this is worth looking into. Here, in a nutshell, is how it works.

Any time you consume food that does not agree with you, your body mounts an inflammatory reaction. It is actually a built-in 'protective mechanism' against the offensive food. Your very cells (all trillion of them) blow up. As a result, you might gain as much as 3-5 pounds overnight!

Continuing to put inflammatory foods into the body produces an ongoing inflammatory state that can build up and create all manner of chronic disease: arthritis, cardiovascular and arterial disorders, immune dysfunction, allergies. And the more inflamed the body becomes, the more foods become reactive to the body.

The typical American diet is **packed full of inflammatory foods** and Americans are living inflamed. The fat patterns that we see, the classic beer belly, excessive abdominal girth, and fat localized to the hips are all signs of chronic inflammation unchecked. This is a fat-adapted body that is begging for attention and relief from the assault of inflammatory triggers.

Other signs can include unexplained illness, maladapted function in multiple systems, and overall malaise. That is, you feel bad and neither you nor your doctor can really figure out why. Given enough time, the chronic inflammation can lead to chronic disease.

The good news? By eliminating inflammatory food, your body has the ability to bounce back and **eventually heal.** And this process can even be relatively quick if you do it right.

Even more exciting than that, given enough time, some of those foods may become less reactive or inflammatory. Some people may be able to go back to those foods after the inflammation settles down.

The truth is, you may not want to go back as your body heals! You will feel so much better that there will be very little motivation to go back to the inflammatory lifestyle.

10

Variety is the Spice of Life

We were created to **enjoy variety**. Our bodies function better when we don't get stuck in nutritional ruts. Actually, the human body thrives on variety. Yes. *Thrives.*

Remember those inflammatory reactions from the last chapter that we can develop to certain foods? One of the reasons we react to certain foods is simply because we are eating too much of *the same thing*...**all the time.**

Not only do **we avoid inflammatory reactions** to food, but **metabolism is also stirred up** by eating a healthy variety of foods. That means taking in a healthy mix of fruits, veggies, and lean meats prepared in new and unusual ways. This, rather than the same mind-numbing, boring rotation of the things *we have learned to like.*

It is really all about 'learning to like' different tastes and *actually enjoying* the variety. On purpose. As a child, my parents were very committed to teaching me the importance of trying different foods. And although some of the things we ate at that time were not stellar nutritionally, the principle of variety was a very sound one, and one that has stood the test of time.

We have learned that eating the same things over and over again **causes your metabolic rate to drop.** Like any other repetitious habit,

your body adapts to eating the same food, so it doesn't take a lot of energy to do the job of digestion.

I encourage you to *broaden your horizons* and **get cooking**. There is absolutely nothin mundane about dining in. Staying home is more economical and being adventurous with your cooking is a wonderful way to expand your palate. So get in that kitchen and create something that is both exciting *and* delectable. Spending more time at home is one of the most lovely gifts that you can give yourself and your family! Enjoy the 'dining in' experience to its fullest by venturing out of your nutritional comfort zone, right in the comfort of your own home!

This does not have to be hard. You can keep it as simple or make it as complex as you like. I love simplicity, but just as variety is the spice of life, spices are a great way to give life to your food and body. Take a look at spices such as cinnamon, turmeric, cardamom, garlic, basil, and cumin.

Cinnamon has been shown to **reduce blood pressure** and along with **turmeric, cumin and cardamom,** has **anti-inflammatory properties. Garlic** and **basil** both have **powerful immune benefits** and many spices are thermogenic. That is, they stimulate fat-burning. Not to mention the addition of extraordinary taste, of course, which will boost your metabolism.

Think of all spices as a **metabolic boost** simply because you are changing it up. So, use them liberally and see what you come up with.

Some final thoughts as we wrap up.

Life is way too short to spend it eating, preparing and planning your food. If you are finding that food is consuming your every thought, you are planning your day around your meals, or you can't

THE HABITS HANDBOOK

seem to get out of the kitchen, please know that all these habits **can change.** You don't have to continue on that path for another minute. You can make whatever change you want to make...right now.

We often over-complicate the whole thing, which actually makes it harder to change. Here are some basic tips to get you moving.

1. Begin with the **end in mind.** Picture yourself in the life you want to have, then craft that life with the decisions you make today and every day.

2. It really only takes **one decision** to make a change in the direction of your dreams. Then one more. And then another. You *can* do this! While it may seem like an impossible mountain to scale, I promise you every mountain expedition begins with one small step. Likewise, every positive change you make starts with one simple step.

3. **Don't deprive yourself.** But at the same time, remember, you don't have to eat the whole pie to enjoy the treat. In fact, it is more of a treat when you don't eat the whole thing. Savoring those tiny tastes of things is often enough. Little samples, fun little bites. Then move on. Go do something. Have some non-food related fun. There is plenty of that out there.

4. Branch out, enjoy your food, give yourself plenty of breaks between meals and then sit back and watch your body heal itself, lean and strong, just the way God intended you to be.

5. **Stop beating yourself up over this.** Stop taking yourself so seriously.

Yes, work as though it all depends on you, but don't berate yourself, mentally flog yourself or otherwise abuse yourself over all the things that you aren't doing as well as you like. This is a literal lifelong pursuit, it is not a race and there really is no finish line. Take your time, learn how to enjoy your food and feel good about all the good you are doing for you!

Lighten up…quite literally!

CONCLUSION

Thank you so much for reading! If you made it here, I could not be prouder of you!

This is not intended to be a comprehensive diet or weight loss course, but merely a set of guidelines that have been proven to work. Not just once. Not just for me. But, over and over again, over many years, across all walks of life. I encourage you to try on the principles and **see how they work for you**.

Remember, even the best advice falls flat if it's not followed..but making even the smallest changes consistently, will trigger a huge cascade of positive changes in the future. One thing I have noticed is that there is a *miraculous momentum* that happens.

When we start to eat better, we have **more energy** and we actually want to move more. The longer you eat better, the less those pesky junk foods appeal to you. You end up in an **upward spiral** that will take you to places you never thought possible. **You will be amazed** at what your body will do for you!

It would give me the greatest joy to know what you are doing with what you have learned here. If you are putting things in place and enjoying the benefits of a healthier body, please share your story!

You can reach me through my website at **www.drlaurasparks.com I would love to hear from you.**

ABOUT THE AUTHOR

Dr. Laura has been a practicing Chiropractor since 1993. She has a passion to see the world healthier by allowing the miraculous healing power of the body to simply do its work.

She is an avid runner, reader and active blogger. Dr. Laura practices all the things that teaches with consistent results. Not only that, but has seen the same results with hundreds of patients. You can find her on FaceBook at Dr. Laura Sparks, on her website at www.drlaurasparks.com or tuning into the Love Your Fit podcast.

This is her third book.